A Paleo Halloween:

Recipes for Your Costumed Cavemen Kids.

Introduction

I want to thank you and congratulate you for downloading the book, "*A Paleo Halloween: Recipes for Your Costumed Cavemen Kids*".

You're about to read great idea for making this Halloween a fun and healthy time your neighborhood kids won't be quick to forget!

Thanks again for downloading this book, I hope you enjoy it!

This document is geared towards providing exact and reliable information in regards to the topic and issue covered. The publication is sold with the idea that the publisher is not required to render accounting, officially permitted, or otherwise, qualified services. If advice is necessary, legal or professional, a practiced individual in the profession should be ordered.

- From a Declaration of Principles which was accepted and approved equally by a Committee of the American Bar Association and a Committee of Publishers and Associations.

The information provided herein is stated to be truthful and consistent, in that any liability, in terms of inattention or otherwise, by any usage or abuse of any policies, processes, or directions contained within is the solitary and utter

Pulsing Pumpkin Soup

This is a crowd pleaser! Best served in small cups so that the neighborhood young ones can easily drink!

Ingredients:

2 tbsp coconut oil

1 chopped onion

1 minced garlic clove

1.5 lb roughly chopped pumpkin flesh

2 medium peeled and roughly chopped sweet potatoes

4 cups fresh chicken stock

1 cup full-fat coconut milk

nutmeg and cinnamon spices

Directions:

Heat a large pot, melt the coconut oil and cook the onion until soft. Add the garlic and cook for one minute.

Add the chopped pumpkin and sweet potatoes and cook for 5 minutes.

Add the stock and sprinkle in salt and pepper. Bring to a boil and simmer for 25 minutes until pumpkin and potatoes are soft to touch.

Stir in the coconut milk and puree with your blender.

Add a dash of cinnamon and nutmeg.

Serve in a small cup to your guests.

Grizzly Ridge Popcorn Balls

The perfect munch and crunch for the little paleo ones in your life this Halloween!

Ingredients:

1 cup honey

1/3 cup light molasses

1/3 cup water

1 tablespoon paleo butter

3 quarts air popped popcorn

medium saucepan

candy thermometer

large bowl

Directions:

Combine honey, molasses, and water in a saucepan.

Cook slowly over medium heat. Stir constantly under the temp on your candy thermometer reaches 250 degrees.

Add in paleo butter and stir in until melted.

Place popped popcorn in a large bowl. Evenly pour syrup over the popcorn and mix well with a spoon.

Let syrup cool and form popcorn into balls with butter greased hands.

Pass them out all night long!

It's scary how much your paleo guest will enjoy snacking on these!

Ingredients:

1/2 cup coconut manna (warmed slightly)

4 tbsp honey

1 pinch of sea salt

1/2 tsp vanilla extract

raisins

mini chocolate chips

parchment paper lined tray to fit in freezer

Directions:

Stir all ingredients together, no including the raisins and chocolate chips. Once mixture is doughy then take a chunk and roll into the size of a large grape. Flatten the sphere out and pinch mini ghost shoes out using your fingertips. Use 2 chocolate chips for eyes and 1 raisin for the mouth. Place tray in freezer to allow them to firm.

Note:

This recipe makes 6 individual Ghost Gobblers so plan accordingly and increase ingredients if needed.

Paleo Zombie Eyes

Delicious and chewy, you won't be running away from these treats!

Ingredients:

1 cup almond flour

1 cup sunflower seed butter

1 tbsp honey

2 tsp vanilla

2 tsp coconut oil

1 cup chocolate chips

Directions:

Combine all your ingredients excluding the coconut oil and chocolate chips.

Form mixture into small spheres or "zombie eyes" and place on wax paper covered cookie sheet.

Allow to harden by placing in freezer for 1 hour.

Melt coconut oil and chocolate chips in a small saucepan over low heat. Keep stirring as now to burn the mixture.

Use a toothpick to carefully dip each sphere 3/4 into the chocolate mixture but making sure to leave a small part uncovered on the top.

Place the "zombie eyes" back into the freezer so they can harden.

Serve when hardened.

Peppermint Patty Wolf Tracks

This recipe will serve 24 of your hungriest paleo guests!

Ingredients:

2 tbsp coconut oil

1 tbsp palm oil

1/4 cup honey

1/4 tsp peppermint oil

1 tsp coconut flour (extra fine)

1 1/4 cup chocolate chips

3 tsp coconut oil

Directions:

Combine coconut oil and palm oil in a small bowl and beat with a hand blender until a creamy like consistency. Then add the honey and peppermint oil and beat again until just as creamy. Set in fridge to chill and thicken up. Form 24 patties the size of a nickel and let harden again in the fridge.

Have a mini muffin pan prepared with liners for later.

Put chocolate chips and coconut oil in a microwave style bowl and microwave in 30 second durations until chocolate is melted. Pour enough of this chocolate in each muffin liner in order to just cover the bottom. Put muffin tin in the fridge to firm up the chocolate.

Once chocolate is firm in the muffin liners you can place a dollop of filling into each liner. Pour chocolate on top of that patty filling and let this all firm up by returning to fridge.

These will be gone soon, I guarantee it!

Frankenstein's Paleo PB Cups

This serves 24 of your little monsters!

Ingredients:

1 cup sunflower seed oil

1/2 cup coconut oil (make sure it's softened)

1/2 cup honey

1/2 tsp vanilla

1/2 tsp salt

1 cup dark chocolate chips

Directions:

Take all ingredients excluding the chocolate and blend in a mixer until smooth.

Melt the chocolate chips in a microwave.

Have a muffin tin prepared with liners (size is up to you, depending on if you want to make small or large PB cups.)

Pour a tbsp of melted chocolate into muffin liners being sure to also coat the sides of the liners with chocolate as well.

Fill with the sunflower mixture and place in the freezer to harden up.

Your little Frankies are going to be talking about these all the way to next year!

Ingredients:

16 ounces of dried apricots

1 cup chocolate chips

1/2 cup chopped pistachios

Directions:

Melt the chocolate chips using microwave or stove.

Dip each apricot halfway into the melted chocolate, then dip into the chopped nuts.

Spread out each apricot on a plate to dry for 30 minutes.

A chewy great Paleo snack!

Ingredients:

1/2 cup coconut butter (warm so it is liquid)

1/2 cup pumpkin puree

1/4 cup coconut oil (warm so it is liquid)

3 tbsp honey

1/2 tsp ground cinnamon

1/4 tsp ground nutmeg

a pinch of salt

6 ounces of dark chocolate

Directions:

Stir together all ingredients, except for chocolate, in a small bowl. Put mixture in fridge so as to make it firm enough to form into small balls.

Form the filling into small spheres which will be the center of the pumpkin patch chocos. Places sphere into fridge to allow them all to become firm.

Melt chocolate in microwave safe bowl. Using a fork you can then dip the filling balls into the chocolate so as to coat them generously.

Place balls on parchment paper line tray and let them cool and firm up before serving.

Ingredients:

24 strawberries

2 cups brown sugar

1 cup coconut milk

1 tbsp coconut oil

1/2 tsp sea salt

1/2 cup chopped pistachio

Directions:

Cook sugar and milk in a saucepan over medium heat. Stir well to dissolve sugar. Turn to low heat and cook for 12 minutes until the liquid turns amber and will coat your spoon.

Add coconut cream, coconut oil and salt. Remove from heat.

Spread chopped pistachio onto plate.

Dip strawberries in salted caramel sauce and then roll in chopped nuts.

Refrigerate for 1/2 hour and serve!

Undead Chocolate Bars

Ingredients:

2 cups unsweetened shredded coconut

1/2 cup honey

1/4 cup melted coconut oil

2 tsp vanilla extract

1/4 tsp salt

chocolate chips

2 tbsp of unsweetened non dairy milk

Directions:

Combine shredded coconut and salt in a food processor until smooth. Put mixture into greased muffin tin.

Combine chocolate chips and milk and heat on stove until melted. Spread mixture on top of coconut filling in muffin tin.

Place cups in freeze and let set and harden before enjoying!

Conclusion

Thank you again for downloading this book!

I hope this book was able to help you to feed your neighborhood kids in a healthy way.

Finally, if you enjoyed this book, then I'd like to ask you for a favor, would you be kind enough to leave a review for this book on Amazon? It'd be greatly appreciated!

www.ingramcontent.com/pod-product-compliance
Lightning Source LLC
Chambersburg PA
CBHW062034280526
45787CB00005B/2313